Horace Wells
On Nitrous Oxide

Thomas Gamsjäger

First Edition 2013
Copyright © Thomas Gamsjäger
CreateSpace Independent Publishing
ISBN-13: 978-1493660230

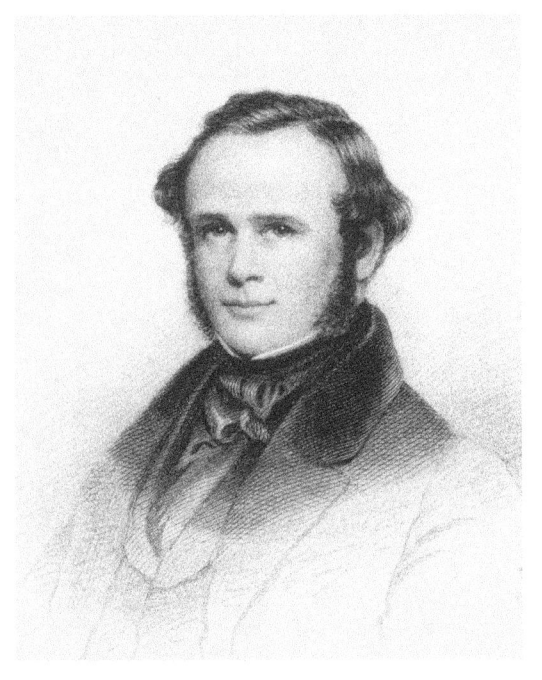

Contents

Introduction 7
Reprint 11
    History of the Discovery of the Application of Nitrous
    Oxide Gas, Ether, and Other Vapors, to Surgical Operations 13
        Preface 15
        History 17
        Testimony 27
Notes on the Sources 41
Bibliography 43
Further Reading 45
Index 47

1

Introduction

Dentist, inventor. But most of all, Horace Wells was a tragic figure. On 21 January 1815 he was born into a comparatively wealthy family in Hartford, Connecticut. He attended the best schools available, and already during his adolescence he was known for his 'restlessness, activity, and intelligence' with repeated praise for his 'inventive genius and great mechanical talent'. Aged 19, he moved to Boston to take up dentistry, which at this time was still more a trade than a profession.[1,2] Why, of all things, dentistry? The historical records still do not give any indication.

After his apprenticeship he went back to Hartford and opened an office on Main Street. The business developed reasonably well, even the Governor of Connecticut, William W. Ellsworth, was among his patients. In addition, he was able to take on students himself. One of them was William T. Morton.[3]

In December 1844 Wells watched the 'Grand Exhibition of the Effects Produced by Inhaling Nitrous Oxide, Exhilarating or Laughing Gas', which was presented by the itinerant lecturer Gardner Quincy Colton. Under the influence of inhaled nitrous oxide one of the participants bruised his leg severely but appeared to feel no pain whatsoever.[4,5,6,7,8] Immediately Wells saw the possible implications of this observation. He might be able to alleviate the sometimes excruciating pain patients had to suffer under his own hands in dentistry. Already on the next day Wells tried the gas himself and had a tooth extracted that had bothered him for quite a while. And he felt no pain! It was 11 December 1844, Nitrous Oxide Day.[9]

Encouraged by the experience, Wells applied nitrous oxide to several of his dentistry patients with resounding success. Therefore, he decided to present his findings to the appropriate representatives of medical profession. But as the occasion arrived when he was granted the opportunity to use nitrous oxide in a tooth extraction in the Massachusetts General Hospital he removed the gas bag to soon, the patient groaned under the pain, and Wells presentation was pronounced 'a humbug affair'.[10,11]

What followed in the ensuing years was a bitter controversy with his former student William T. Morton. Morton was the first to use ether as an inhalational anaesthetic in 1846, but he claimed the whole concept of inhalational anaesthesia as his own development without acknowledging Wells' discovery with respect to nitrous oxide from two years before.[12]

Wells was not able to counter Morton's often unscrupulous handling of the matter. Embittered he more or less gave up dentistry, but he tried to continue his work on anaesthetics in the course of which he heavily self-experimented with chloroform. In a psychologically deranged state he attacked two women in the open street which brought him to New York's Tombs Prison. There, on 24 January 1848 he committed suicide, at the age of only 33.[13]

---

[1] Archer, *Life and Letters*, pp. 83-84.
[2] Ellsworth, *Life of Horace Wells*. In: Smith, *An Inquiry into the Origin of Modern Anaesthesia*, pp. 8-9.
[3] Archer, *Life and Letters*, pp. 89-99.
[4] Archer, *Life and Letters*, p. 177.
[5] Smith and Hirsh, *Gardner Quincy Colton*, pp. 383-384.
[6] Archer, *Life and Letters*, p. 107.

7   Colton, *Anaesthesia. Who made and developed this great discovery?*, pp. 4-5.
8   Colton, *A True History of the Discovery of Anaesthesia*, pp. 3-4.
9   Colton, *A True History of the Discovery of Anaesthesia*, pp. 3-4.
10 Archer, *Life and Letters*, p. 109.
11 Archer, *Life and Letters*, pp. 119-121.
12 Archer, *Life and Letters*, pp. 131-134.
13 Archer, *Life and Letters*, pp. 136-142.

2

Reprint

The following section represents a reprint[1] of one of Horace Wells' few writings[2], a small pamphlet entitled 'History of the Discovery of the Application of Nitrous Oxide Gas, Ether, and Other Vapors, to Surgical Operations', which was published in 1847 by J. Gaylord Wells in Hartford, Connecticut. In essence, in a somewhat haphazard way Wells addresses the scientific community and the wider public supported by numerous testimonials in order to establish what seemed to him to be his due right, his priority in the discovery of nitrous oxide as an inhalational anaesthetic.

---

[1] The spelling of the original text is unchanged, only minor adaptations have been made with regard to punctuation to aid readability.
[2] The only other relevant publication is his book 'An Essay on Teeth; Comprising a Brief Description of their Formation, Diseases, and Proper Treatment' of 1838.

Horace Wells

History of the Discovery of the Application of Nitrous Oxide Gas, Ether, and Other Vapors, to Surgical Operations

Preface

In answer to a request, made by several scientific and medical societies of Europe, who have desired me to furnish them with the evidence of my priority of discovery of the application of gas, or vapor, for the performance of surgical operations, I have obtained testimonials and affidavits sufficiently numerous and satisfactory, as I believe, to establish the fact beyond a doubt. I have forwarded the original papers to Dr. C. S. Brewster of Paris (No. 11 Rue de la Paix), who will have charge of them until this question is settled.

The following pages contain a correct copy of those papers, which prove, conclusively, that I made known this discovery in November, 1844, which date is nearly two years prior to that given by Drs. Jackson and Morton.

Horace Wells

Hartford, March 30, 1847

History

To the European and American Public:

I propose, in the briefest manner possible, to give, in the following pages, a true and faithful history of the discovery which is at present causing an unparalleled excitement throughout the whole medical world. I refer to the administering of exhilarating gas, or vapor, to prevent pain in surgical operations. It is very unfortunate that there should be more than one claimant for the honor of the discovery; but so it is: and the only alternative now is, for the man who considers himself entitled to this honor to present his proofs, that a discriminating and impartial public may "give credit to whom credit is due".

Reasoning from analogy, I was led to believe that surgical operations might be performed without pain, by the fact, that an individual, when much excited from ordinary causes, may receive severe wounds without manifesting the least pain; as, for instance, the man who is engaged in combat may have a limb severed from his body, after which he testifies, that it was attended with no pain at the time; and so the man who is intoxicated with spirituous liquor may be severely beaten without his manifesting pain, and his frame, in this state, seems to be more tenacious of life than under ordinary circumstances. By these facts I was led to enquire if the same result would not follow by the inhalation of exhilarating gas, the effects of which would pass off immediately, leaving the system none the worse for its use. I accordingly procured some nitrous oxide gas, resolving to make the first experiment on myself, by having a tooth extracted, which was done without any painful sensations. I then performed the same operation for twelve or fifteen others, with the like results.

This was in the fall of 1844. Being a resident of Hartford, Connecticut, I proceeded to Boston, in December of the same year, in order to present my discovery to the medical faculty; first making it known to Drs. Warren, Hayward, Jackson, and Morton; the last two of whom expressed themselves in the disbelief that surgical operations could be performed without pain, both admitting that this modus operandi was entirely new to them; and these are the individuals who now claim to be the discoverers!

By invitation of Dr. Warren, I addressed his medical class upon the subject. I embraced the opportunity, and endeavored to establish the principle that the system, when wrought up to a certain degree of nervous excitement, by any means whatever, would thus be rendered insensible to pain, and would admit of surgical operations being performed without any disagreeable sensations. In proof of this theory, I related my experience in extracting teeth under the influence of nitrous oxide gas, stating that, with one or two exceptions, all on whom I had operated (numbering twelve or fifteen) assured me that they experienced no pain whatever; and, in further proof of the truth of this principle, I cited analogous cases, as, the man who is excited by passion, or he who is much intoxicated by liquor; stating, that individuals under these circumstances uniformly testify, when wounded, that such injuries were inflicted without pain. I stated, also, that I was making use of nitrous oxide gas simply because I considered it more harmless than any thing else which could be used for this purpose; assuring them that the same result would follow, let the nervous system be excited sufficiently in any manner whatever. I remained several days in Boston in order to have an opportunity of administering the gas to a man who was expecting to have a limb amputated, but the operation was postponed. I was then invited to extract a tooth for a patient in presence of the medical class, which operation was performed, but not with entire success, as the gas-bag was removed too soon; and as the man said he experienced some pain, the whole was denounced as an imposition, and no one was inclined to assist me in further experiments.

The excitement of this adventure immediately brought on an illness, from which I did not recover for many months; being thus obliged to relinquish, entirely, my professional business. I will now, in a few words, state how the names of Jackson and Morton came into notice, as being connected with this discovery.

Dr. Morton, who is a dentist in Boston, was instructed in his profession by myself, about five years since, and I subsequently assisted in establishing him in the city of Boston, and after I had made the above discovery, I had frequent interviews with him; and he, being aware that I had relinquished my professional business in consequence of a protracted indisposition, requested me to instruct him how to prepare the gas which I had been giving so successfully in Hartford, stating that he wished to make a trial of it in Boston. As this interview was in Hartford, I told him to request Dr. Charles T. Jackson (with whom we were both acquainted) to prepare him some of it, as he was a chemist. Accordingly, Dr. Morton went to Dr. Jackson for the gas, who gave him the ether, as being attended with the least trouble. After one or two teeth were extracted, it was then introduced into the Massachusetts General Hospital, where a capital operation was performed under its influence with perfect success; which fact was immediately published in the principal newspapers of the day, with the names of Jackson and Morton (who had, by a written contract, entered into a sort of co-partnership business in this matter) as the discoverers; and Dr. Jackson, as I have since been informed, immediately sent letters to London and Paris, to be read to the several Academies, where he takes all the credit to himself, not even mentioning the name of Morton, his partner by written contract, which contract was signed and executed on the 27th of October, 1846. In this agreement, Dr. Jackson acknowledges that

Dr. Morton made the discovery "in conjunction" with himself, as the following extract from the paper signed by Jackson fully proves:

> "To all persons to whom these presents shall come: Whereas, I, Charles T. Jackson, of Boston, in the State of Massachusetts, chemist, have, in conjunction with William T. G. Morton, of said city, dentist, invented, or discovered, a new and useful improvement in surgical operations on animals, whereby we are enabled to accomplish many, if not all operations, such as are usually attended with more or less pain and suffering, without any, or with very little, pain or muscular action, to persons who undergo the same," etc.

After the fact came to the knowledge of Morton that Jackson had sent privately to Paris, he, as a natural consequence, became very indignant; and each of these individuals now deny that the other has had anything to do with the discovery which was at first claimed by both, "acting in conjunction." I will here make a quotation from the Boston Advertiser, of March 6th, 1847, which contains Dr. Morton's reply to Dr. Jackson. Dr. Morton proceeds as follows:

> "In the letter to M. Beaumont, of Paris, from which I have already made extracts. Dr. Jackson says:
>
> 'Five or six years ago, I remarked the peculiar state of insensibility into which the nervous system was plunged by the inhalation of the vapor of pure sulphuric ether,' etc.
>
> Previously to this, he had already stated, under oath, in the preamble to the specifications, which bear date the 27th of October, 1846, that the same hath not, to the best of his knowledge and belief, been previously known. Now, Dr. Jackson either did know, previous to this time, that sulphuric ether would produce insensibility to pain, or he did not. If he did as stated in his letter to M. Beaumont, then I have to remind him of his oath, under the solemnity of which he states that, according to the best

of his knowledge and belief, 'the fact had not been before known.' But if he did not, then I remind him of his statement to M. Beaumont, in which he says that he had known it for 'five or six years.' And the learned Doctor may take either horn of the dilemma he may prefer.

It is not known that Dr. Jackson ever made more than one experiment in inhaling ether; and then he used it as an antidote to the vapor of chlorine, which he had accidentally breathed, but from his own statement, in the Advertiser, it did not answer the purpose – the deleterious effects returning with the return of consciousness. But, supposing he had known of it six years or six months before Dr. Morton applied it in practice, is it not inexcusable in him to have withheld from suffering humanity this inestimable boon so long – a boon by the gift of which such an incalculable an amount of misery might have been saved? Or is it within the limits of probability, that if he had been so long in possession of a discovery which, if made known, would in four months call down blessings on his head from ten thousand hearts, and from all civilized lands, and which, from present prospects, would make him to be remembered and cherished by the side of Jenner by all coming generations, and to all coming time – I say, is it probable, had he known of this noble gift, that he would not have been more zealous in publishing it to the world? If he did make this discovery, is it not a remarkable coincidence that Dr. Morton should have made it at the same time, and still more remarkable, that Dr. J. should leave to another the honor to make his discovery known? But to settle this whole matter, and it might have been done in the outset, to the satisfaction of any candid mind: After Dr. Morton began to use the ether in his practice, and for some weeks, it is well known to a large number of our most respectable citizens, that Dr. Jackson clearly and distinctly repudiated and washed his hands of the whole thing. He, on many occasions, as it is well known to his friends, disclaimed all connection with the discovery or use of ether in surgery. A gentleman of high standing, asked Dr. J., in presence of several others, if he 'knew that, by the inhalation of ether, such a state of insensibility could be produced as that the knife could be applied, and the patient feel no pain?' Dr. J. replied: 'No; nor Morton either, nor any one else. It is a humbug, and it is reckless in Morton to use it as he does.'

In speaking to two other persons, at different times, on this subject, he said: 'I don't care what he [Morton] does with it [the discovery], if he does not drag my name in with it.'

At another time, he said, he 'did not know how it would work in pulling teeth, but he knew its effects at college upon the students, when the faculty had to get a certificate from a physician that it was injurious, to prevent them from using it.' Many other statements, on this point, can be given, but it is deemed wholly unnecessary. The above, and other statements even stronger, can be verified by affidavits."

When it was announced in the Boston papers that Drs. Jackson and Morton claimed this discovery, the citizens of Hartford were taken by surprise, for it was well known here that I had put in practice the same more than two years before, and not only this, but it was generally known that I had long since made a journey to Boston exclusively on this business, in order to present it to the medical faculty. Dr. P. W. Ellsworth, a son of the Hon. W. W. Ellsworth, Ex-Governor of Connecticut, who was acquainted with the circumstances above mentioned, immediately published an article in the Boston Medical and Surgical Journal, stating those facts that came under his personal observation – which accord perfectly with what I have already stated. Dr. E. E. Marcy, of this city, also published an article in the Journal of Commerce about the same time, stating that he was knowing to my making the discovery, and going to Boston in 1844, when I had an interview with Dr. Jackson, who said that he did not believe that surgical operations could be performed without pain, when I informed him of the discovery I had made. Dr. Marcy quoted Dr. Jackson's language to me, and in his (Jackson's) reply, he does not deny that I had this interview with him, but simply says that he did not use the words which are credited to him in the quotation marks. He does not deny but that the substance of those words were said by him; and, furthermore, he cannot deny this.

This letter of Dr. Jackson, in reply to Dr. Marcy, requires still further notice. He says that he had merely heard that I had tried some experiments with nitrous oxide gas, but had never heard that they were successful. Now I am fully persuaded that Dr. Jackson does not remember the circumstance of his being informed and assured in November, 1844, that my operations were uniformly successful, with but one or two exceptions; but such was the case, and the individual who informed him of this fact will make the statement under oath, if necessary. Dr. Jackson was then informed that I had operated on twelve or fifteen patients by the use of nitrous oxide gas, without causing the least pain, in but two instances.

Dr. Jackson claims that the nitrous oxide gas and the vapor of ether are essentially different in their effects when inhaled. He asserts, in this letter, that sulphuric ether, as it is used in Boston, does not act as a stimulant, but has the reverse effect. In reply to this statement. Dr. Marcy quotes an article from the Boston Medical and Surgical Journal, where Dr. J. C. Warren, of the Hospital, in his report, proves that ether, as given in Boston, acts as a stimulant; but in order to prove, even to the satisfaction of Dr. Jackson himself, that he was mistaken, I will quote his own language, from an article published in the Boston Advertiser, of March 8, 1847. He says:

> "We are aware that ether ranks in the pharmaceutic books and dispensatories, as a diffusible stimulant, and that its fumes or vapor produce intoxication of short duration."

The fact is, that nitrous oxide gas and the vapor of ether, are identical in their effects; first exhilarating, then, when continued to excess, the reverse effect follows, acting as a sedative, throwing the person into a deep sleep or stupor.

This discovery does not consist in the use of any one specific gas or vapor, for anything which will cause a certain degree of nervous excitement, is all that is required to render the system insensible to pain; consequently, the only question to be settled is, which exhilarating agent is least likely to do harm? I have confined myself to the use of nitrous oxide gas, because I became fully satisfied, from the first, that it is less injurious to the system than ether. In the fall of 1844, after I had tried several experiments with nitrous oxide gas with perfect success – then wishing to use a substitute which would be attended with less trouble in its preparation – I advised with Dr. E. E. Marcy, of this city, at which time we discussed the comparative merits of nitrous oxide gas and rectified sulphuric ether. Knowing that both had the same effects upon the system, so far as causing insensibility to pain was concerned, the object of the discussion was to ascertain which would do least harm. I had, previous to this, inhaled ether, as well as nitrous oxide gas, and found their effects upon the nervous system to be precisely the same; but I found it very difficult to inhale the vapor of ether in consequence of the choking sensation. For this reason, and for the reason that Dr. Marcy and myself came to the conclusion that nitrous oxide gas was not so liable to do injury, I resolved to adhere to this alone. Let it be observed, however, that at this time (November, 1844), while we had the subject under consideration, a surgical operation was performed at Dr. Marcy's office, under the influence of sulphuric ether, as is proved by affidavit. The Doctor then advised me, by all means, to continue the use of nitrous oxide gas.

If the question is asked, why so much time has elapsed since its first discovery, without its coming into more general use, I can only say, that I have used my utmost endeavors, from the first, to influence physicians and surgeons to make a trial of it, assuring them that my operations were numerous, and perfectfully successful. But all were fearful of doing some serious injury with it; and not wishing to incur the responsibility of administering this powerful agent without the co-operation of the medical faculty, and also for the reason that I was obliged to relinquish my professional business in consequence of ill health, my operations have been somewhat limited.

On making the discovery, I was so much elated respecting it, that I expended my money freely, and devoted my whole time for several weeks, in order to present it to those who were best qualified to investigate and decide upon its merits, not asking or expecting any thing for my services, well assured that it was a valuable discovery. I was desirous that it should be as free as the air we breathe; but judge of my surprise, after the lapse of many months, when I was informed that two individuals (Drs. Jackson and Morton) had claimed the discovery, and had made application for a patent in their own names.

After making the above statement, and submitting the following testimonials and affidavits, I leave it for the public to decide to whom belongs the credit of this discovery.

Respectfully,

Horace Wells

Testimony

Boston, March 23, 1847

We, the undersigned, residents of Boston, Mass., testify, that in the fall of the year 1844, while attending lectures given by Dr. J. C. Warren, of the Massachusetts General Hospital, the students were informed by Dr. Warren, at the close of his lecture, that Mr. Wells, of Connecticut, was present, and would address them upon the subject of rendering the system insensible to pain, during the performance of surgical operations, by the inhalation of exhilarating gas. The students accordingly retired to an adjoining room, where we were addressed upon this subject by Mr. Horace Wells, of Hartford, Conn., who invited us to meet in the evening to witness an operation, which operation was performed in our presence, while the patient was under the influence of the gas.

THOMAS WM. KENNEDY, M. D.
Office corner of North Charles and Livingston Streets, Boston
P. B. MIGNAULT, M. D.

City of Boston: On this 23d day of March, A. D. 1847, the above-named Thomas J. W. Kennnedy, M. D., and P. B. Mignault, M. D., personally appeared before me, the subscriber, Mayor of the city of Boston, and made oath that the above certificate, by them subscribed, is true.

In testimony whereof I subscribed the same and caused the city seal to be hereunto affixed, the day and year last within written.
JOSIAH QUINCY
Mayor of the city of Boston, Justice of the Peace

Hartford, March 26th, 1847
I, the undersigned, resident of Hartford, Connecticut, testify, that, in the fall of the year 1844, while attending medical lectures, given by Dr. John C. Warren, of the Massachusetts General Hospital, the students were informed by Dr. Warren, at the close of his lecture, that Mr. Wells, of Connecticut, was present, and would address them upon the subject of rendering the system insensible to pain during the performance of surgical operations, by the inhalation of exhilarating gas. The students accordingly retired to an adjoining room, where we were addressed upon this subject by Mr. Horace Wells, of Hartford, Connecticut, who invited us to meet in the evening to witness an operation, which operation was performed in our presence, while the patient was under the influence of the gas.
CINCINNATUS A. TAFT, M. D.

State of Connecticut,
Hartford County, ss:
City of Hartford, March 27, 1847
Then personally appeared before me, Cincinnatus A. Taft, who signed the foregoing affidavit, and made solemn oath that the same was true.
Given under my hand and the seal of said city.
A. M. COLLINS, Mayor

Boston, March 23, 1847

I hereby certify, that the following gentlemen attended my Lectures on Anatomy and Surgery in the season of 1844-45, viz: Thomas Wm. Kennedy, P. B. Mignault, and Cincinnatus A. Taft.

JOHN C. WARREN

Professor of Anatomy and Surgery

Boston, March 23d, 1847

I do hereby testify that Horace Wells, of Hartford, Connecticut, with whom I have been acquainted for several years, came to Boston in the year 1844, (I think in November or December) and informed me that he had made a valuable discovery, which enabled him and others to perform surgical operations without pain. He then informed me of the result of his experiments, which he assured me were numerous, and perfectly successful. I accompanied him to a hall in Washington street, where a large number of medical students had assembled, as I understood, to witness an operation to be performed by Dr. H. Wells, upon a patient while under the influence of exhilarating gas, which was the discovery above referred to. The gas was administered, and the tooth extracted under its influence by the said Wells, in presence of myself and many others. I am not able to say whether the patient experienced any pain or not. There was certainly no manifestation of it, yet some present expressed themselves in the belief that it was an imposition.

I was subsequently informed that his operations in Hartford, prior to 1845, were uniformly successful under the influence of gas.

DANIEL T. CURTIS

No. 23 Bedford street

City of Boston: On the twenty-third day of March, A. D. 1847, the above-named Daniel T. Curtis, personally appeared before me, the subscriber, Mayor of Boston, and made oath, that the foregoing certificate, by him subscribed, is true.

In testimony whereof I have subscribed the same, and caused the city seal to be hereunto affixed, the day and year last above written.

JOSIAH QUINCY

Mayor of the city of Boston, Justice of the Peace

I hereby certify, that Horace Wells, dentist, has, for more than two years, had the reputation, in this city, of having made a discovery which enabled him, and others, to extract teeth without pain, by the use of exhilarating gas. I have conversed with several gentlemen, whose reputation for honor and veracity places them above suspicion, who have had these operations performed by the said Wells, in the fall of 1844 ; and they assure me that the operation was attended with no pain whatever. There is no doubt in my mind that said Wells discovered and made the first practical application of this principle in surgical operations. By comparing dates of the several claimants, there can remain no doubt of this fact.

S. FULLER, M. D.

Hartford, March 25th, 1847

Hartford, March 25, 1847

As attempts have been made to deprive Mr. Horace Wells, dentist, of the honor of discovering the effects produced by certain gases in allaying pain, I feel it my duty to state the facts in the case. Dr. Jackson does not claim an earlier discovery than the latter part of

1846, and even then only suggested to Mr. Morton that ether might answer the purpose, and says that the first trials of Morton were successful, "proving exactly as I had predicted." The first trial of Morton, according to his own (Morton's) statement, was on the 30th Sept., 1846. Now, I hereby declare, that to my full knowledge, nitrous oxide gas was administered two years earlier than this, viz., in 1844, by Mr. Wells, and that many teeth were extracted without pain under its influence; and that Mr. Wells went to Boston at that time, as I was then informed, for the purpose of introducing the gas to the attention of surgeons in that city. Moreover, in an article published June 18th, 1845, in the Boston Medical and Surgical Journal, I referred to it as a thing well known and established – the article being headed, "On the Modus Operandi of Medicine," written to show that many, if not all, local diseases, are cured by specific stimulants. Now, when it is known that Mr. Morton was instructed in his profession by Mr. Wells, and introduced into business by him, we can easily trace the manner in which Mr. M. might have derived his information. It is to be borne in mind, also, that Jackson and Morton have, through the public prints, each denied the other his claim – a thing easily settled, one would think, if it in justice belonged to either. In my own mind, there is not a shadow of doubt that the whole merit of the discovery of this thing rests with Wells, and with him alone, although others may have experimented with ether before him. The idea and its practical application are his, and let the public concede that to him which his generosity, unrestricted with patents, demands, and which has been, as far as possible, wrested from him. The claimants in Boston I do not know, and should be unwilling, in any manner, to injure their feelings, but I must say that they are laboring under an hallucination at least; though I cannot but hope they may be able to establish some claim to originality – a task somewhat difficult, as the case appears to stand. These statements are given, not from any personal considerations, but simply as an act of justice; and I hope that the profession, after due deliberation, will give a righteous award.

P. W. ELLSWORTH, M. D.

I take pleasure in certifying, that more than two years since, at the request of Horace Wells, Esq., of this city, I visited his rooms for the purpose of witnessing the extraction of a tooth from a man, while under the influence of the nitrous oxide gas. The idea was novel to me, and I took occasion to be present during the operation. The gas was administered by Mr. Wells, and the operation performed without any apparent suffering on the part of the individual operated upon. I afterwards questioned him in regard to his sensations during the extraction, and he assured me that he had not experienced the slightest degree of pain. At this time, the comparative merits of the gas and of rectified sulphuric ether vapor, were discussed, and I gave it as my opinion, that the nitrous oxide gas was the safest, inasmuch as the after-effects of this gas are not so unpleasant as from the ether vapor. I also take this occasion to assert, from my positive knowledge, that the ether vapor was administered very soon after this period (and prior to 1845) for the performance of a surgical operation.

In conclusion, I beg leave to offer it as my opinion, that the man who first discovered the fact that the inhalation of a gaseous substance would render the body insensible to pain, during surgical operations, should be entitled to all the credit or emolument which may accrue from the use of any substances of this nature. This is the principle – this is the fact – this is the discovery. The mere substitution of ether vapor, or any other article, for the gas, no more entitles one to the claim of a discovery than the substitution of coal for wood in generating steam, would entitle one to be called the discoverer of the powers of steam.

E. E. MARCY, M. D.

Hartford, March 27th, 1847.

State of Connecticut,
Hartford County, ss:
City of Hartford, March 27, 1847
Personally appeared E. E. Marcy, Physician and Surgeon, resident in this city, and made solemn oath to the truth of the foregoing affidavit by him subscribed before me.
Given under my hand and the seal of said city, the day and year aforesaid.
A. M. COLLINS, Mayor

This is to certify, that during the last two or three years, I have been familiar with the successful operations of Mr. Horace Wells, and other dentists of this city, in extracting teeth, without pain, by the aid of nitrous oxide gas, and he, alone, was regarded as the author of this discovery.

G. B. HAWLEY, M. D.

Hartford, March 27th, 1847

I, John M. Riggs, surgeon dentist, of the city and county of Hartford, State of Connecticut, in the United States of America, being of lawful age, and duly sworn, do depose and say:

That on or about the first of November, Anno Domini one

thousand eight hundred and forty-four, I was consulted by Horace Wells, surgeon dentist, of the city, county and state as aforesaid, as to the practicability of administering nitrous oxide gas prior to the performance of dental or surgical operations.

Thinking favorably of the suggestion, it was decided to make trial of the gas in question; and on the day following, per agreement, the protoxide of nitrogen was administered to Horace Wells, aforesaid, at his request, and I extracted one of his superior molar teeth: he manifesting no signs of suffering, and stating that he felt no pain during the operation.

Encouraged, and gratified with the success of the first experiment, the aforesaid Wells and myself continued to administer to various individuals the said gas, and to extract teeth while under its influence, in the presence of several gentlemen, until fully satisfied of its usefulness and applicability in surgical operations. I further affirm that the said Wells avowed his intention to communicate the discovery to the dental and medical faculty, and, in pursuance of that intention, proceeded to the city of Boston, State of Massachusetts, for that purpose; whilst I continued to use the said gas with great success – the patients assuring me they felt no pain.

JOHN M. RIGGS

State of Connecticut,
Hartford County, ss:
City of Hartford, March 27, 1847
Personally appeared John M. Riggs, and made solemn oath to the truth of the foregoing affidavit, by him subscribed before me. Given under my hand, and the seal of said city, the day and year above written.
Given under my hand and the seal of said city.
A. M. COLLINS, Mayor

I, the undersigned, resident of Hartford, Connecticut, do hereby testify, that, more than two years since, I submitted to the operation of having a tooth extracted while under the influence of nitrous oxide gas. According to the best of my recollection, this was in the month of November, 1844. The gas was given, and the tooth extracted by Horace Wells, dentist, of Hartford; and I do further testify that the operation was attended with no pain whatever.
MYLO LEE.

State of Connecticut,
Hartford County, ss:
City of Hartford, March 26, 1847
Then personally appeared before me, Mylo Lee, signer of the foregoing affidavit, and made solemn oath that the same was true. Given under my hand, and the seal of said city.
A. M. COLLINS, Mayor

During the winter of 1844, I learned that Dr. H. Wells, dentist, Hartford, Conn., had discovered the mode of extracting teeth without pain. This was accomplished by administering to the persons operated upon exhilarating gas or vapor, which, it was asserted, rendered the human system insensible to pain. At first I was incredulous of the fact, and received the assertions of individuals familiar with the operation with a degree of distrust. Being, however, by invitation, a personal witness of the process of extracting teeth without pain, under this new mode, discovered and practiced by Dr. Wells with so much apparent success, I was induced to submit to a personal operation, that I might test its utility. The Dr. was most successful – extracting for me a large, firmly-set bicuspid tooth, without the slightest sensation of pain.

I also witnessed, soon after, a repetition of the same process, by Dr. Wells, upon several individuals, accompanied, in every instance, with perfect success.

F. C. GOODRICH
Hartford, March 27, 1847

State of Connecticut,
Hartford County, ss:
City of Hartford, March 27, 1847
Then personally appeared before me, F. C. Goodrich, of this city, who signed the foregoing affidavit, and made solemn oath that the same was true.
Given under my hand and the seal of said City.
A. M. COLLINS, Mayor

Hartford, March 26, 1847
I hereby testify, that, more than two years prior to this date, on being informed that Horace Wells, dentist, of this city, had made a valuable discovery, by which means he could extract teeth without pain to the patient, which consisted in the use of stimulating gas, or vapor, I inhaled the exhilarating gas, and, under its influence, had six extracted without the least pain. I would further state, that for more than eighteen months from the time I first submitted to this operation by the application of gas, I heard no other name mentioned as the discoverer, except that of the above-named Horace Wells.

J. GAYLORD WELLS
184 1/2 Main street

State of Connecticut,
Hartford County, ss:
City of Hartford, March 26, 1847
Then personally appeared before me J. Gaylord Wells, of this city, who signed the within deposition, and made solemn oath that the same was true.
Given under my hand, and the seal of said city.
A. M. COLLINS, Mayor

A little more than two years since, I learned that Dr. H. Wells, dentist, of this city, had made the discovery that by the use of an exhilarating gas or vapor, he could render the nervous system insensible to pain under severe surgical operations, and that he was using it in his practice with success. Having an opportunity to witness its effect upon several persons, during the operation of extracting teeth, I was so delighted and surprised with its manifest success, that I desired a trial of it upon myself. The gas was accordingly administered, and two carious teeth were extracted from my lower jaw, without the least suffering on my part; though ordinarily, owing to the firmness with which my teeth are fixed in my jaw, I suffer extreme pain from their extraction.
WM. H. BURLEIGH
Editor of the "Charter Oak"
Hartford, March 25, 1847

State of Connecticut,
Hartford County, ss:
City of Hartford, March 26, 1847
Then personally appeared before me, William H. Burleigh, signer of

the foregoing affidavit, and made solemn affirmation that the same is true.

Given under my hand and the seal of said city.

A. M. COLLINS, Mayor

To whomsoever it may concern:

We, the undersigned, physicians of the city of Hartford State of Connecticut, U. S. A., do hereby certify, that we know, and have conversed with the persons whose names are appended to the above affidavits, viz., Wm. H. Burleigh, J. G. Wells, F. C. Goodrich, Mylo Lee, and place implicit reliance upon the statements made therein, by each of them, to wit: that the operation of extracting one or more teeth without producing any pain, whatever, was performed upon each of them, by Horace Wells, surgeon dentist, of this city, at or about the time specified by them respectively, in their several affidavits above referred to.

We take pleasure, also, in expressing our entire confidence in the integrity of the said Horace Wells, than whom no person in our city is more favorably known, as a gentleman of honor and integrity. We know, moreover, that he has for several years past successfully devoted himself to subjects pertaining to invention and discovery.

S. FULLER, M. D.
GEORGE SUMNER, M. D.
BENJ. ROGERS, M. D.
J. B. BERESFORD, M. D.
H. ALLEN GRANT, M. D.
WM. JAMES BARRY, M. D.
E. E. MARCY, M. D.
C. A. TAFT, M, D.
DAVID S. DODGE, M. D.
P. W. ELLSWORTH, M. D.

GURDON W. RUSSELL, M. D.
G. B. HAWLEY, M. D.
E. K. HUNT, M. D.
DAVID CRARY, M. D.
JOHN SCHUE, M. D.
HENRY LEE, M. D.

I certify that the foregoing document is subscribed by the principal surgeons and physicians of the city of Hartford, in the State of Connecticut, U. S. A.
ISAAC TOUCEY
Hartford, March 29th, 1847

State of Connecticut, ss:
Office of Secretary of State.
I hereby certify, that his Excellency Isaac Toucey, (whose name, in his own handwriting, is subscribed to the foregoing certificate,) is Governor in and over the State aforesaid.
In testimony whereof, I have hereunto set my hand and affixed the seal of said State, at Hartford, this 29th day of March, A. D. 1847, and in the 71st year of the Independence of the United States of America.
CHARLES WM. BRADLEY
Secretary of State

3

Notes on the Sources

The full bibliographic information on this reprint:

Author	Horace Wells
Title	History of the Discovery of the Application of Nitrous Oxide Gas, Ether, and Other Vapors, to Surgical Operations
Year of publication	1847
Publisher	J. Gaylord Wells, Hartford

The steel engraving on page 3 is attributed to H. B. Hall.

The artist who created the miniature painting on page 49 is unknown.

4

Bibliography

Archer, W. Harry. *The Life and Letters of Horace Wells, Discoverer of Anesthesia*. Kessinger Legacy Reprints 2010

Colton, Gardner Quincy. *Anaesthesia. Who made and developed this great discovery?* A. G. Sherwood, New York 1886

Colton, Gardner Quincy. *A True History of the Discovery of Anaesthesia*. A. G. Sherwood, New York 1896

Smith, Gary B.; Hirsh, Nicholas P. *Gardner Quincy Colton: Pioneer of Nitrous Oxide Anesthesia*. Anesth Analg 1991; 72: 382-391

Smith, Truman. *An inquiry into the origin of modern anaesthesia*. Brown and Gross, Hartford 1867

Wells, Horace. *An Essay on Teeth; Comprising a Brief Description of their Formation, Diseases, and Proper Treatment*. Case, Tiffany & Co, Hartford 1838

5

Further Reading

Fenster, Julie M. *Ether Day*. Perennial, New York 2002

Index

anaesthetic, inhalational 8

Barry, Dr. 38
Beaumont, M. 20
Beresford, Dr. 38
Boston 7, 18, 19
Boston Advertiser 20, 23
Boston Medical and Surgical Journal
.... 22, 23, 31
Bradley, C. Wm. 39
Brewster, Dr. 15
Burleigh, Wm. H. 37, 38

chlorine 21
chloroform 8
Collins, A. M. 28, 33, 34, 35, 36, 37, 38
Colton, G. Q. 7
Crary, Dr. 39
Curtis, Daniel T. 29

dentistry 7
Dodge, Dr. 38

Ellsworth, Dr. 22, 32, 38
Ellsworth, W. W. 7, 22
Essay on Teeth 11
ether 19, 20, 21, 23, 24, 31, 32
exhilarating gas 17

Fuller, Dr. 38
Fuller, S. 30

Goodrich, F. C. 36
Grand Exhibition 7
Grant, Dr. 38

Hartford 7, 18, 22
Hawley, Dr. 33, 39
Hayward, Dr. 18
Hunt, Dr. 39

Jackson, Dr. 15, 18, 19, 22, 25, 30
Journal of Commerce 22

Kennedy, Thomas Wm. 27

Lee, Dr. 39

Lee, M. 35
limb amputation 18

Marcy, Dr. 22, 23, 24, 33, 38
Massachusetts General Hospital...8, 19, 27, 28
Mignault, P. B. 27
Morton, Dr. ...7, 15, 18, 19, 22, 25, 31

New York 8
Nitrous Oxide Day 8

operations, surgical 17

priority 15

Quincy, J. 28, 30

Riggs, J. M. 33
Rogers, Dr. 38
Russell, Dr. 39

Schue, Dr. 39
Sumner, Dr. 38

Taft, Cincinnatus A. 28
Taft, Dr. 38
Tombs Prison 8
tooth extraction 17
Toucey, I. 39
Warren, Dr. 18, 23, 27, 28, 29
Wells, J. Gaylord 36, 41

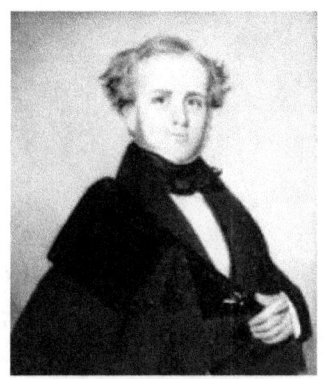

www.ingramcontent.com/pod-product-compliance
Lightning Source LLC
Chambersburg PA
CBHW071827170526
45167CB00003B/1445